Essential Oils:

50 Best Essential Oil Recipes -
Discover The Magic Power Of
Essential Oils And Natural
Remedies For Abundant Health,
Beauty And Longevity!

I0420666

Table of Contents

Introduction

Essential oils can be traced back in history to around 1550 BC. This is quite a long time, but the ancient people knew that essential oils have a wide variety of benefits. Essential oils can beaten, put on the skin, diffused, and even placed in a bath.

They can help with anything from stress to even being in your bathroom routine. Since they have a wide variety of uses you can place them in your life for almost anything, here you'll find some ways to improve your health, beauty, and longevity.

Chapter one will go through a variety of ways to help improve your health with the use of essential oils. Removing chemicals from your health improvement will increase your overall health because you're not putting something potentially harmful into your body.

Essential oils have been used for centuries to help improve the health of the individual. Essential oils have been shown to boost immunity, reduce blood pressure, heal bug bites and sunburns, and even help to heal athlete's foot.

You can also remove some of the pills you take now for certain things, like allergies.

Anything homemade is usually better for you than store bought, because you don't add the extra additives that the companies do to help preserve the product.

Chapter two will help you remove those pesky chemicals from your beauty routine. There are so many chemicals in beauty products that cause damage to your immune system, brain function, and can cause various cancers. Here you can take your favorite essential oils and make them into shampoos, baby shampoos, perfumes, deodorant, toners, acne remover, shower gels, and even salt scrubs.

By making your favorite products at home you can ensure they smell the way you want them to, and feel the way you want them to. You can also ensure yourself you and your family are using products that are safe for everyone.

Chapter three will help increase your life with mood boosters, anxiety relief, immunity help, emotional healers, allergy relief, and holiday blends as well as set a romantic mood. The longevity that essential oils increase will help you feel better about yourself and those around you.

Longevity is a combination of various things including health and mood. If you have both good health and mood then you're less likely to have bad blood pressure, stress, and anxiety.

No matter what you're looking to do essential oils can help increase any mood. With several ways to use essential oils there is no reason to not use them and improve your life today.

By using these recipes you'll increase your health, beauty, and overall longevity. Let's begin by improving your health with our first chapter.

Chapter 1 – Abundant Health Recipes

There are several ways that essential oils can help with your health. They can alleviate illnesses like athlete's foot, acne, and can even help boost your immunity when you have a cold.

Your health is what keeps your body moving, gives you energy, and just keeps you alive. It is a very important part of your life, and if you're looking for a way to increase your health you're in the right place.

Here are few ways you can improve your health with the help of essential oils.

PMS Bath

Ingredients:

- 3 drops geranium oil
- 4 drops ylang ylang oil
- 4 drops Clary sage oil
- 1 teaspoon massage or olive oil

Instructions:

Fill the bath with warm water and add in all the ingredients. Stir the oils into the water before entering. Soak in the water for about 30 minutes, allowing the aromas from the oils to penetrate your nose.

Bug Bites and Sunburns

Ingredients:

- 4 oz. bottle
- Nature's Fresh
- Powdered vitamin C Ascorbates
- 4 drops lavender oil
- 1 to 2 drops Helichrysum oil

Instructions:

Fill the bottle most of the way with the Nature's Fresh. Add in all the ingredients and shake. Add to your bug bites and sunburns. The Helichrysum oil does not need to be added but it helps relieve pain and increases healing speed. This can be taken on camping and rafting trips to help your spots right away, so make sure your container is easy to take with you.

Immune Booster

Ingredients:

- 40 drops lavender oil
- 20 drops Tea Tree oil
- 10 drops Roman Chamomile oil
- 10 drops lemon oil
- Carrier oil (such as almond or coconut), or massage oil

Instructions:

Mix all the ingredients into whatever air tight container you want. Apply close to the nose so you can inhale the scent. This recipe can also be used in a bath if you choose. You can also place in a diffuser to increase the immunity of everyone in a room. This is especially good for those with multiple kids who always get sick together, one right after the other.

Stuffy Nose

Ingredients:

- 6 drops Eucalyptus oil
- 3 drops lemon oil
- 3 drops Neroli oil

Instructions:

Mix all the oils into your choice container. Apply close to the nose until stuffy nose is gone. This recipe can also be used in the bath or a diffuser, just as long as you inhale the scent.

If you choose to place in a container you can take it with you when you go and have relief on the go.

Blood Pressure Reducer

Ingredients:

- 10 drops lemon oil
- 10 drops sweet marjoram oil
- 10 drops ylang ylang oil
- 30 drops Clary sage oil

Instructions:

Mix all the ingredients together and apply on the skin. The best places are on the bottom of the feet or on the upper chest, near the neck. Apply daily or when you begin to have issues.

Relaxation Inducer

Ingredients:

- 50 drops mandarin oil
- 25 drops lavender oil
- 12 drops sweet marjoram oil
- 5 drops sandalwood oil

Instructions:

Mix all the oils together and apply near the nose. You can also apply on the bottom of the feet. This recipe can be used in a diffuser, and is not recommended for extended baths.

Warning: You may fall asleep in the bath if used for an extended time.

Athlete's Foot

Ingredients:

- 5 drops massage oil
- 2 drops Tea Tree oil
- 1 drop lavender oil

Instructions:

Mix all the ingredients in your hand and massage onto feet and between toes. Wash hands after use. Apply to the feet at least twice a day.

Use until you're Athlete's foot is completely gone.

Premenstrual Cramps

Ingredients:

- 10 drops ylang ylang oil
- 10 drops Clary sage oil
- 10 drops lavender oil

Instructions:

Fill your bathtub with warm water and add in all the oils. Mix the oils before entering. Soak at least once a day when symptoms are present.

Try soaking for about 30 minutes to truly relieve the pain and allow the oils to soak into the skin.

Reduce Binge-Eating

Ingredients:

- 10 drops Clary sage oil
- 10 drops ylang ylang oil

Instructions:

These two oils will boost your self-confidence, making it so you don't want to binge-eat. You can apply this recipe to the bottom of your feet or bathe in it.

It's best used when you have the cravings to eat when you don't need to.

Cold and Flu

Ingredients:

- 10 drops Eucalyptus oil
- 10 drops pine oil

Instructions:

Mix the oils together either in a daily bath or add to a diffuser. This recipe is best inhaled. Place some on your pillow at night where you can smell it as well to help clear up that cold.

Use this recipe until your cold clears up and you feel you no longer need it.

Quit Smoking

Ingredients:

- 10 drops massage or carrier oil (sweet almond or coconut oil)
- 10 drops thyme oil
- 10 drops ylang ylang oil
- 10 drops pine oil

Instructions:

Add the carrier or massage oil to a container. Add in the other oils and stir gently. Rub near your nose and keep excess nearby so you can inhale often. This simulates the smell of smoking so instead of taking in dangerous chemicals you're inhaling something beneficial. This is a great substitute in places where smoking is not permitted. You can add this recipe to a diffuser as well.

Constipation

Ingredients:

- 15 drops rosemary oil
- 10 drops lemon oil
- 5 drops peppermint oil
- 2 tablespoons massage or vegetable oil

Instructions:

Mix the massage oil and the essential oils together. Rub this mixture on your lower abdomen in a counter-clockwise motion. Apply three times a day until constipation clears.

Aching Joints

Ingredients:

- 10 to 20 drops Eucalyptus oil

Instructions:

Fill your tub with warm water and add in the Eucalyptus oil. Stir before entering and soak for about thirty minutes.

Warning: You may fall asleep in the bath if used for an extended time.

Stress Relief

Ingredients:

- 30 drops bergamot oil
- 10 drops geranium oil
- 10 drops ylang ylang oil

Instructions:

Mix all the oils together and either add to a diffuser or rub onto the bottom of the feet.

Ear Infection

Ingredients:

- 1 teaspoon massage oil
- 3 drops Tea Tree oil
- 1 drop thyme oil
- 2 drops lavender oil

Instructions:

Mix together the oils and apply around the ear, down the neck, and across the cheekbone. This follows the path of the infection so it can help clear up the whole thing.

Brain Boost

Ingredients:

- 7 drops massage oil
- 5 drops rosemary oil
- 1 drop peppermint oil

Instructions:

Mix the oils in your hand. Apply around the face, taking care not to get it in your eyes. Also rub on your neck, and if there is any remaining oil left rub into both hands. This will help pep up your brain and give you a boost.

Chapter 2 – Beauty Enhancement Recipes

There are so many beauty products out there, and most of them are filled with harmful chemicals. Have no fear, there is a solution. You can eliminate the chemicals in your beauty routine and come out smelling amazing with essential oils.

The real question you have to ask yourself now is what to do with all those old useless beauty products.

Peppermint Rosemary Shampoo

Ingredients:

- ½ cup castile soap
- ½ cup water
- 16 drops rosemary oil
- 2 drops peppermint oil
- Container with easy open lid

Instructions:

Add the soap to the container. Add in the oils and water last. Gently shake and use as normal shampoo.

Lavender Honey Lip Balm

Ingredients:

- 2 tablespoons coconut oil (unrefined is best)
- 1 tablespoon shea butter
- ½ teaspoon raw honey
- 1 tablespoon sweet almond oil
- 2 tablespoons beeswax
- 15 drops lavender oil
- 5 drops frankincense oil
- 12 empty lip balm containers (or the like)
- A large rubber band

Instructions:

In a double boiler melt the coconut oil, shea butter, honey, and beeswax until nice and smooth. It may become a clear color or be very pale when completely melted. Remove from heat and add in the almond oil and essential oils.

Use the rubber band to hold down the lip balm tubes and pour the liquid into the tubes before they cool. Allow to cool with the lids off until the liquid becomes a cool solid.

Foaming Face Wash

Ingredients:

- ½ teaspoon sweet almond oil
- 1/3 cup castile soap
- 10 drops ylang ylang oil
- 6 drops patchouli oil
- 4 drops lemon grass oil
- 2/3 cup water
- 1 foaming soap dispenser

Instructions:

Pour the castile soap and the almond oil into the dispenser. Add the essential oils and swirl the bottle to combine. Fill the rest of the bottle with water. Use this scrub on your face daily for best results.

Shower Gel

Ingredients:

- 2/3 cup castile soap
- 2 tablespoons raw honey
- 1 teaspoon vitamin E oil
- 1 teaspoon jojoba oil (pronounced hohoba)
- 10 drops ylang ylang oil
- 5 drops Idaho Blue Spruce oil
- 2 teaspoon vegetable glycerin

Instructions:

Wisk together the soap, honey, vitamin E oil, vegetable glycerin, and the essential oils. Place into any container you would want to keep in the shower.

Mint Sea Salt Scrub

Ingredients:

- 1 ½ cups sea salt
- 1/3 cup sweet almond oil or olive oil
- 3 drops peppermint oil
- 3 drops spearmint oil

Instructions:

Mix together the sea salt and the almond oil. Mix together while pouring the almond oil over the salt. Add in the essential oils. Scrub your feet with the scrub and allow them to rest for five minutes. Wash away with warm water and pat your feet dry. Finish by adding your favorite moisturizer.

Green Tea Toner

Ingredients:

- 8 ounce bottle
- ¼ cup brewed organic green tea
- 2 tablespoons apple cider vinegar
- ¼ cup water
- 10 drops frankincense oil
- 10 drops lavender oil

Instructions:

This recipe is great for acne. Simply place all the ingredients into the bottle. Gently shake to mix and apply to trouble areas at least once daily.

Deodorant

Ingredients:

- 2 tablespoons beeswax
- 1 ¼ tablespoon shea butter
- 1 ¼ tablespoon coconut oil
- ½ tablespoon Bentonite clay
- ½ tablespoon baking soda or arrowroot
- 10 drops lemon grass oil
- 6 drops rosemary oil

Instructions:

This deodorant is designed to work for both men and women, so matter who you are you can get rid of chemicals under your armpits. On low heat in a double boiler melt together the beeswax, coconut oil, and shea butter.

Mix well and melt until there are no chunks. Mix in the baking soda (or arrowroot) and the clay. If you move the mixture into a bowl make sure the bowl isn't metal, as Bentonite clay can change the composition of the metal, making it poisonous.

Let the mixture cool for a few minutes then add in the essential oils. Pour the mixture into an old deodorant container with the plunger all the way down.

Let the mixture cool with the cap off until hard. Use like you would any other deodorant.

Whipped Coconut Oil Body Butter

Ingredients:

- ¾ cup coconut oil
- ¾ cup shea butter
- 1 tablespoon jojoba oil
- 1 tablespoon vitamin E oil
- 10 drops lavender oil
- 20 drops orange oil
- 1 teaspoon vanilla extract

Instructions:

In a glass bowl use a hand mixer to blend together the coconut oil and shea butter. Mix on high until they become nice and fluffy. Add the remaining ingredients and whip. Store in an air tight container in a cool dark place.

Body Polish

Ingredients:

- 1 cup white sugar
- ¼ cup honey
- 2 teaspoons jojoba oil
- 1 teaspoon vanilla extract

Instructions:

Combine all the ingredients together and stir until blended well. Store in an air tight container.

Baby Shampoo

Ingredients:

- 1 cup castile soap
- 1 cup coconut oil
- 1 cup water
- 10 drops lavender oil

Instructions:

Use an old plastic bottle and place all the ingredients inside. An old baby shampoo bottle will work well. Use as normal shampoo but rinse immediately after use or baby will look greasy. Their skin will be even softer with this blend and the lavender will help relax them, making this a great shampoo to use before bed time.

Mouthwash

Ingredients:

- 2 teaspoons calcium carbonate powder
- 1 teaspoon xylitol crystals
- 10 drops concentrated trace minerals liquid
- 10 drops peppermint oil
- 5 drops lemon oil
- 5 drops spearmint oil
- 2 cups of water

Instructions:

Mix all the ingredients together and allow the crystals to dissolve. After they are dissolved it is ready to use. Store in the fridge. This will keep in the fridge for up to 2 weeks. This specific recipe helps to re-mineralize your teeth, ridding you of cavities and sensitive spots.

Body Cream

Ingredients:

- 1 cup whipped coconut oil
- ½ cup jojoba oil 5 to 8 drops sweet orange oil (or your choice of essential oils)
- 1 to 2 teaspoons melted beeswax

Instructions:

Use a hand mixer to whip the coconut oil until nice and fluffy. Use a double boiler and melt the beeswax. Combine all the ingredients and blend well. Store in an airtight container.

Citrus Lavender Perfume

Ingredients:

- 2 teaspoons beeswax
- 2 teaspoons sweet almond oil or jojoba oil
- 24 drops lavender oil
- 24 drops sweet orange oil

Instructions:

Mix the essential oils and set aside. Melt the beeswax in a double boiler and add in all the oils. Place into a container of your choice

27

(such as a tin) and let cool. This is a rub on perfume so it will become hard after cooling. These are easy to take perfumes and also make great gifts.

Medicated Lip Balm

Ingredients:

- 2 tablespoons shea butter
- 2 tablespoons beeswax
- 2 tablespoons coconut oil
- 10 drops vitamin E oil
- 10 drops Tea Tree oil

Instructions:

In a double boiler melt together the beeswax and the essential oils. Add in the shea butter and melt until nice and smooth. Should be a good liquid with no lumps.

Remove from heat and pour into any container you like. Let cool with the lid off. When done you now have a lip balm that repairs cracks and puts moister back into your lips.

Also helps to heal other sores on the lips.

Shaving Cream

Ingredients:

- 1/3 cup coconut oil
- ½ cup shea butter
- 1 tablespoon jojoba oil
- 15 drops lavender oil
- 5 drops peppermint oil
- 5 drops eucalyptus oil
- 1 teaspoon baking soda

Instructions:

Melt the coconut and jojoba oils in a double boiler until they become clear. Remove from heat and whisk in the essential oils, baking soda, and shea butter. Refrigerate until the mixture is solid and white. Whip with a hand mixer until nice and fluffy. Place in the fridge for another hour or until the mix resembles heavy cream. Spoon into containers and you're done.

Coconut Body Wash

Ingredients:

- ½ cup coconut milk (get it from the cans not the carton)
- 2/3 cup castile soap
- 3 teaspoons vitamin E oil
- 5 drops of your favorite essential oil(s)
- 2 teaspoons vegetable glycerin

Instructions:

Simply place all the ingredients in your chosen container for the shower, shake, and use. You'll get the great healing power of the vitamin E oil and the smell of coconut and your favorite essential oil smell.

Muscle Relief Cream

Ingredients:

- 6 drops frankincense oil
- 6 drops Tea Tree oil
- 6 drops peppermint oil
- 3 drops clove oil
- 3 teaspoons coconut oil

Instructions:

Place all the ingredients in your chosen container, gently shake to mix. Do not use on sensitive areas, such as genitals or around the eyes. If the mixture is too intense reduce the amount of peppermint oil. This recipe warms the sore muscle to give them pain relief.

Stretch Mark Remover

Ingredients:

- 2 oz. Rosehip seed oil
- 9 drops Neroli oil
- 9 drops lavender oil

Instructions:

Use a dark glass bottle for the storage of this recipe. Add in the Rosehip seed oil to the glass bottle. Add in the essential oils on top. Rub the mixture on your stretch marks daily until the marks are gone. Store in a cool dark place.

Chapter 3 – Longevity Recipes

The overall lifetime of the human being is slowly being cut by chemicals in our products. Wouldn't it be nice to increase your time here on earth?

Well there are several ways that you can increase your longevity. Stress is a big factor in creating health issues. Here are some recipes that you can use to increase your mood and your overall longevity.

Fatigue Helper

Ingredients:

- 4 drops grapefruit oil
- 6 drops peppermint oil
- 5 drops rosemary oil

Instructions:

This recipe is for a diffuser. Just add the oils into the diffuser and turn it on. Breathe in the healing oils and inhale several times to relieve fatigue.

Stress Relief

Ingredients:

- 6 drops lavender oil
- 4 drops Roman chamomile oil
- 4 drops ylang ylang oil

Instructions:

This recipe is for the diffuser. Add the drops to the diffuser and turn on. Breathe in the stress relieving aroma and feel the stress melt away.

Memory Boost

Ingredients:

- 1 drop basil oil
- 1 drop rosemary oil
- 2 drops lemon oil
- 2 drops peppermint oil
- 2 drops grapefruit oil
- 2 drops lavender oil

Instructions:

This recipe is for a diffuser. Add the oils into the diffuser and turn on. Allow the smell to be inhaled a few times before you require that extra brain power. You'll feel your brain being stimulated after a couple times inhaling.

Anxiety

Ingredients:

- 5 drops lavender oil
- 5 drops lime oil
- 5 drops mandarin oil

Instructions:

This recipe is for the diffuser. Add the oils to the diffuse and turn it on. Inhale and feel the anxiety leave you.

Immunity

Ingredients:

- 6 drops lemon oil
- 5 drops grapefruit oil
- 5 drops orange oil

Instructions:

This recipe is for the diffuser. Add the oils to the diffuser and turn on. This best used for when you have a cold or feel one coming on. It will help you fight off the germs and increase your overall health.

Energy

Ingredients:

- 2 ounces of carrier oil (sweet almond, coconut oil, and so forth)
- 6 drops Clary sage oil
- 15 drops lavender oil
- 10 drops lemon oil

Instructions:

Mix all your oils in your chosen container and gently shake to stir. Apply this recipe to the bottom of your feet or near your nose. You'll feel a pep in your step a few minutes after application.

Focus

Ingredients:

- 2 ounces of carrier oil (sweet almond, coconut oil)
- 12 drops basil oil
- 12 drops lemon oil
- 8 drops rosemary oil

Instructions:

If you're looking for a recipe that will increase your focus look no further. Add all the ingredients in a container of your choice and apply on the bottom of your feet or near your nose. After application it will feel like a wakeup call. Do not overuse, or it will lose its potency.

Topical Immunity

Ingredients:

- 2 ounces carrier oil (sweet almond, coconut oil)
- 10 drops geranium oil
- 10 drops lavender oil
- 10 drops vetiver oil

Instructions:

Mix all the ingredients in your choice container. Apply this to the bottom of your feet whenever you feel your need it. If you have a cold place some on your pillow where you can smell it. You can also take this on the go to apply whenever you like.

Anti-stress

Ingredients:

- 2 ounces carrier oil (almond oil, coconut oil)
- 5 drops Neroli oil
- 8 drops nutmeg oil
- 17 drops petigrain oil

Instructions:

Mix all the oils in your choice container. Apply to the bottom of the feet or near the nose. Apply when you begin to feel stressed.

Daily Blend

Ingredients:

- 15 ml bottle
- 10 drops orange oil
- 8 drops frankincense oil
- 8 drops bergamot oil
- 1 drop Neroli oil
- 3 drops Roman Chamomile oil
- 4 drops cypress oil
- 2 drops vetiver oil
- 1 drop clove oil

Instructions:

Put all the oils into the bottle. Do not shake the contents, but roll to mix up the oils. Apply to the bottom of the feet daily to achieve best results. This recipe helps reduce stress, lifts the mood, and helps reduce blood pressure. This is the best daily recipe to apply to promote longevity, as it covers almost everything.

Emotional Healing

Ingredients:

- 2 drops wild orange oil
- 2 drops bergamot oil
- 2 drops cypress oil
- 2 drops frankincense oil

Instructions:

If you've been having some problems emotionally whether it's being upset or even depressed then this is the recipe for you. You can place this recipe in a diffuser or a bath. It will elevate your mood, allowing you to think clearly about your other emotions and solve your problem. This is a great recipe if you're a bath person, because you can relax as well as heal yourself emotionally.

Allergy Away

Ingredients:

- 2 drops peppermint oil
- 2 drops lemon oil
- 2 drops lavender oil

Instructions:

You can place this recipe in a diffuser or apply near the nose. The smell helps relieve allergy symptoms, so take it when you feel the symptoms. Taking some to apply topically will help you reduce the use of allergy pills and the like.

Mental Clarity

Ingredients:

- 2 drops frankincense
- 2 drops vetiver oil
- 4 drops Garden Align or Balance

Instructions:

Mix the oils together and apply on the bottom of the feet. Within minutes you're be thinking more clearly than before. You can also place this recipe in the diffuser to fill your whole room or home with the smells of clarity. Make sure not to use too frequently, or it will lose the effect.

Workout Blend

Ingredients:

- 8 drops grapefruit oil
- 4 drops lavender oil
- 4 drops lemon oil
- 2 drops basil oil

Instructions:

Mix all the ingredients into your chosen container. Apply to the bottom of your feet about ten minutes before a workout. You'll feel more motivated to workout than before and have the energy to make it through to the end.

Romantic Mood

Ingredients:

- 7 to 10 drops sandalwood oil
- 2 drops vanilla oil
- 1 drop jasmine or ylang ylang oil

Instructions:

If you're looking for a way to set a romantic mood for you and your partner then look no further. Place this recipe in a diffuser to spread it around the house for a night of spontaneity. Use this for date night or if you're just looking to surprise that special someone.

Holiday Bliss

Ingredients:

- 4 to 6 drops patchouli oil
- 2 to 4 drops cinnamon oil
- 3 to 5 drops sweet orange oil
- 1 to 2 drops clove oil
- 1 drop ylang ylang oil

Instructions:

The smells of the holidays are one of the most favorite things about them. Now you have a recipe to invoke that holiday smell whenever you want. Place all the ingredients in a diffuser to spread around your home. You can place this on your body as a perfume as well, but don't put too much on or it will be overbearing.

Conclusion

Well, there you have it. Some 50 recipes that you can use to eliminate chemicals from all sorts of products as well as get the benefits of using essential oils.

Centuries have passed and the benefits of these essential oils has not changed, and even now we understand them even better.

So no matter how you choose to use the essential oils you will receive everything you expect from them, aromatherapy, health resolutions, and even mood boosters.

Essential oils can help with your health issues, no matter what they are. If you want to relieve stress, use some lavender. Make sure to have a carrier oil like almond oil or coconut oil for some of the recipes that require them.

These oils help with the smells of the essential oils and how quickly they evaporate on your skin. If you're looking for just healthy tips then keep eucalyptus oil and Tea Tree oil around, as quite a few recipes call for one or the other.

Health wise essential oils can help with anything from cramps, muscle pains, stuffy noses, bug bites, sun burns, and can even reduce blood pressure. If you could reduce the amount of pills you have to take just by using essential oils, would you do it?

Beauty products are used by both men and women, and eliminating those products you use now filled with chemicals for the ones that call for essential oils may save you from future health risks. Beauty products are filled with chemicals that have shown to cause cancers and other diseases.

These beauty products do call for things other than essential oils, and you should be able to find them on a co-op, or you can easily buy them online.

Buying a product in store however gives you a chance to read the label as well as judge how big you'll need the product to be.

Here we have everything from shampoo, body scrub, shower gel, shaving cream, lip balm, and even homemade deodorant. With a little patience and practice you'll have these beauty products in your home with no problems.

They even make great gifts for those in your family who enjoy homemade gifts. Who doesn't like getting something homemade for free?

Increasing your overall longevity includes several things, such as, increasing your health and mood.

The recipes here are mainly for mood boosters. Those who are less stressed have been shown to have less heart problems or bad blood pressure issues.

Included in these is immunity boosters, anxiety relief, memory boost, energy increase, and even a blend that will motivate you to workout...because we all like to put things like that off, don't we?

Longevity is the length of our lives, and increasing this with essential oils will not only make your life longer but you'll have a better, more boosted life.